I0423155

BOB HOFFMAN'S SIMPLIFIED SYSTEM OF BARBELL TRAINING

(Original Version, Restored)

by

BOB HOFFMAN

Olympic Coach

Originally Published in 1942

PUBLISHED BY O'Faolain Patriot L L C, Copyright 2012

info@physicalculturebooks.com

ISBN-13: 9781475015942

ISBN-10: 1475015941

Published in the United States of America

To Order More Copies Visit:
PhysicalCultureBooks.com

The information contained in this publication is for historical and educational purposes only and is not designed to and does not provide medical, nutritional, or health advice, diagnosis, or opinion for any health or individual problem. The material presented is not a substitute for medical or other professional health services from a qualified health care provider who is familiar with the unique facts of the individual, and should not be used in place of a visit, call, consultation, or advice of a physician or other healthcare provider. Individuals should always consult a qualified health care provider about any health concern and prior to undertaking any new treatment. The publisher assumes no responsibility and specifically disclaims all liability for any consequence relating directly or indirectly to any action or inaction that a reader takes based on any information contained herein.

Be advised that no one should undertake exercises in the nature of those addressed in this book without prior consultation with a physician. Nor does the publisher make any representations concerning whether any of the exercises or suggestions provided by the trainers or physical fitness specialists featured in this book would be effective or appropriate for the reader's needs or expectations. The publisher expressly disclaims any and all responsibility and/or liabilities that might result from the uninformed or misinformed application of the techniques identified herein as well as for any unsupervised physical fitness training.

Finally, the publisher disclaims any and all liabilities arising from the use of any equipment featured in this book and makes no representations as to the utility, safety, or adequacy of the equipment generally or with respect to any specific purpose.

A Word About the Author

Born Nov. 9th. 1898. Tifton. Ga. Weight 8 pounds. Paternal grandparents. Swiss-English. Maternal grandparents, Scotch-Irish.

1901—Narrowly escaped death from typhoid fever, said to have weak heart.

1902—Showed first interest in athletics by excelling other boys running round tennis court 200 times.

1903—Started school two months before 5th birthday.

1909—At age of ten won modified marathon race of ten miles for boys under 16.

1910—Followed his first "train you by mall" Physical Culture course. The Swoboda system.

1911—Moved to West Virginia, grew up along Ohio River—learned to swim, puddle, row, skate, fish, hunt, trap and greatly enjoyed all outdoor activities.

1912—First reached his present height of 6ft 3 in., weight 140 pounds, mostly legs.

1913—Played football on Ohio valley team, against men nearly twice his age, some of whom became great All-American players a bit later.

1914—Moved to Pittsburgh, graduated from high school—went to work as shipping clerk, to earn money to go to college. Continued interest in athletics by spending spare time on river, canoeing and swimming.

1915—Won the national championship, quarter mile canoe race as well as many other prizes at aquatic sports.

1916—Repeated win of national championship, competed in thirteen events in one regatta, winning not worse than third in any of them—thirteen silver cups in all—was named the "iron man" by the Pittsburgh newspapers.

1916—Had worked during summer vacation on dams, construction jobs, this year worked in factory making shells for British government—went to work at Spaldings Athletic Store a few months later—soon leading sales through great interest in and knowledge of athletics of all sorts. By this time had won hundreds of trophies of all sorts, medals, watches, plaques, cups, as well as numerous championships.

1917—'The war year: enlisted two days after war was declared. 6 weeks later selected to go to officers' training school at Fort Niagara, N.Y.. Was leading the class, when it was discovered that Bob was only 18. Law that officers must be 21 years of age. Went back to his organisation. Was soon a sergeant, trained at Augusta, Ga, in preparation for the trip to Franco. Was in charge of physical training in his regiment, excelled at all forms of athletics in the army, won first the regimental boxing championship, then was divisional and corps champion. Had weighed 167 pounds in the athletic activities of 1910. Finally weighed a bit over 175, so was the heavy-weight champion of his part of the army. Won the national championship as well as other events while on army leave.

1918— Early in the year went to France— was member of Co. A 111th Infantry. 28th Penna. division. Before the actual fighting he fought British champions Bandsman Rice and Bombardier Wells, the French champion George Carpentier, the navy and marine champions, including Gene Tunney, as well as many U. S. Army champions. In June moved to the front, was selected as one of the first to fight, distinguished himself in first action by capturing 38 prisoners, after 12 bullets had left their mark on his body or equipment. Back to the hospital and then to the front again. During this year took part in all the major battles of the American Army, was gassed and decorated time after time. His list of decorations include: Belgian Order of Leopold, highest Belgian decoration, Italian War Cross, French Croix de Guerre with palms and stars, American order of the Purple Heart, Silver Star medal for extreme gallantry in action, Special Distinguished Service Medal and D. S. C. After the armistice, continued with army athletics, receiving his officer's commission by special congregational action late in 1918, just before his 20th birthday.

1919—Home in August, won the national championship in canoeing his first day at home and other first prizes. Continued with athletics.

1920—Made another step toward his present work by taking a job, selling a book on health and exercise, called the Library of Health, one thousand pages, price $20.00, moved to York, Penna.

1921 to 1927—Continued at work in manufacturing business, finally rose to the presidency of the company, continued interest in physical training in spite of unusual volume of work.

1923—Finally learned the apparently carefully guarded secret that all strong men had trained with barbells. To this point all his athletic training, all his practice with mail order courses and all forms of exercise, had built his weight to just 170 after the fighting in France, to 180 in this year of 1923. Was not particularly strong, and could not properly press 80 pounds when he first tried the barbell, after considerable effort put up 50 pounds with one hand.

1924—After one year of irregular barbell training due to pressure of business, had gained to 191 pounds, won a contest to find the strongest man in York with lifts of 150 bent press, 140 one hand clean and jerk, 135 two hands snatch, 185 clean and jerk, 417 dead weight lift.

1925—Learned that barbell training had greatly improved his athletic ability at all sports, won 44 medals on one business trip by competing in every form of athletics in which there was competition in the cities he visited during this trip of 6 weeks' duration— mostly aquatics, swimming, rowing, canoeing, but also shot putting, running, broad jump, boxing and wrestling.

1926—Rowed as a member of an eight oar championship crew in Philadelphia.

1927—Won every event In which he had an opportunity to compete. District boxing and wrestling crowns, hexathlon championship, national heavyweight weight lifting championship, county quoit pitching championship, hand boll championship, etc., etc., etc. Moderate barbell training and lifting made it possible for Bob to excel at every physical activity. It gave him power, speed, co-ordination, timing, judgment of space and distance so that he could control the little rubber ball in hand ball, the three pound quoit with tosses of 40 feet, played 212 games in the country championships and leading up to them without a single defeat and at the same time lift heavy weights. Convinced a great many people that weight training was the best form of conditioning.

1928-1929-Early-1930—Devoted major time to business, constantly travelling, driving model T Ford 50,000 miles a year, carrying 105 pound barbell as part of his baggage, kept in good shape and competed when he could.

1930—Went back into weight lifting competition, one of the place winners in the senior national championship that year, the first York barbell, still in daily action, had been built. This is the bell that Bob used to establish his modern world's record of 282 in the one hand lift over-head (bent press style). The famous York team had its beginning that year. Soon was seeking and obtaining matches with all the teams in the east.

1931—The York team got better and better, was nearing the top.

1932—Strength and Health magazine, of which Bob Hoffman has been the editor from beginning to now, had its inception. Four York lifters made the Olympic team. Bob had been selected as trainer of the Olympic team. York team first won national team title which it has held to present, four Yorkers won national titles this year.

1933—Bob won professional lifting championship of America, in competition, heavyweight class. Completed his famous twenty weeks of training, during which he established world's records in physical gains and lifting ability. At the completion of this program, weighed 243½ pounds. He proved the York System to be the world's best physical training system.

The years passed. In 1938 Bob was trainer for the American Olympic team again. York team had gone up, Terlazzo winning the Olympic championship. Each year from this point on members of the York team won greater honors, for several years holding all the U. S. records in the three lifts and totals, establishing most of the world's records, winning many world's titles. Bob grew bigger and stronger, weighing 205 pounds recently. Although 50 pounds was all he could put overhead one hand in the beginning in spite of years of intensive athletics, on his 38th birthday, Bob first lifted 202 pounds overhead with one arm. On his 39th-220, his 40th-263½, his 41st-270, his 42nd-275, his 43rd-282.

Bob Hoffman had an ordinary beginning physically, he proved his interest in and knowledge of athletics in winning well over 500 athletic trophies, he has proved his knowledge of body building by reaching the top of the physical training world, he's the world's leading physical director, the author of a dozen popular books, editor of "Strength and Health" magazine, the world's leading physical training magazine. When you follow one of his courses you can be sure that you follow the best instruction which can be had. Bob is your instructor, your counsellor. With your effort, using York barbells and following his instruction, he guarantees your success.

Everybody Should Exercise

YOU are about to launch on what has proven to be the very best form of physical training. While the chief object of barbell physical training is to aid the individual who practices such exercises to keep fit in the shortest possible period of time, with the least expenditure of energy, barbells have long proven their ability to produce the maximum of strength and development. Every strong man worthy of the name has trained considerably with barbells. To obtain strength and muscle, with resulting development, the muscles must be made to work. The harder the work, the greater the results obtained. All the best built men who take part in the Mr. America contest, or the many preliminary Best Built Man contests which lead up to the great national event, practice with barbells.

While few men or women who follow the simplified system of barbell training offered in this course desire great strength or large muscles, the graduates of the school of strength and health, the barbell way, have proven that this system is best. York has long been famed as the center of the strength world. Members of the York Barbell Club year after year win all or nearly all of the national weight lifting titles, invariably the other places are won by York trained men. All the United States records and the majority of the world's records are held by members of the York team. All proof that we know our business and that Bob Hoffman's York courses of training are soundly and scientifically arranged and do bring superior results.

As we will constantly reiterate throughout this course, you obtain from exercise what you put into it, the champions of strength and development put all they had into barbell training. They became the world's strongest and best built men. If you wish to reach the limit in strength, health and development, after following these courses for a time, you will desire more weight and more equipment. The addition of the famous York 7 in 1 outfit will provide you with adjustable dum- bells, York patented Health Shoe and Head Strap.

But if your wish is only to keep superlatively fit, strong both inside and out, following this course which is known as Bob Hoffman's Simplified System of Barbell Physical Training will bring you the results you desire. Practicing the same proven to be best system of training, which has produced scores of thousands of superbly built and powerful men, handling less weight, and practicing for shorter training periods will bring you as much of the champions' strength and development as you wish to attain.

Progressive barbell training was practiced by the ancient Chinese, Japanese, Hindus and Egyptians. Milo of Crotona, who gained endless fame as the strongest man of his time, trained progressively as he carried the small calf each day until it grew to be a huge bull. This was an early example of progressive training. In this country, for at least a century, weights have been employed by those who sought more than average strength. In 1902, a barbell system was offered for sale by a subsidiary of the York Barbell Company. More than a decade ago a greatly improved, more result producing system of barbell training was offered to the strength and health seeking world by Bob Hoffman. It quickly proved its superiority over all others and rapidly forged to the front, thus becoming the world leader. Over two hundred thousand York barbells are in use throughout the world. This system consisted of four courses of exercises, weight lifting movements and the practice of actual weight lifting. The usual training equipment included a 210 pound barbell, dumbell bars, head strap, wrist developer, York Iron Boots, with the addition of a dumbell course consisting of 48 exercises and a leg course of 20 additional exercises.

This set of weights, the equipment and courses it contained, proved itself to be the best system of physical training. It still is the very best, but considerable lime is required to use the various appliances which make up the famous Bob Hoffman's "Big Twelve Special." Sufficient space is required for the use of the longer bar, to prevent many persons, who should benefit from this form of training, from exercising in their homes with barbells.

For this and a host of other reasons, one of which was the desire to develop a system of training which would make it possible for large groups of men to train in a minimum of time with barbells, this new and simplified system of barbell training was devised. While it will bring favorable, even startling results, it will not completely supersede the heavier, more complete sets of weights, and the additional courses. Rather we hope and expect that it will be a means of introducing this best form of physical training to hundreds of thousands or millions of additional men and women.

Everyone who desires physical betterment, to feel well and to look well, can experience the unusually favorable results of barbell training, now that this simplified system, this new and beautiful barbell with its time saving features, can be had. This streamlined, simplified system of barbell training devised by Bob Hoffman, the world's leading physical director, will provide the maximum of benefit, in the minimum of time. The moderate cost of the equipment, the small space required for this modern form of barbell training, makes it possible for every intelligent man or woman to taste the thrilling benefits of weight training.

Lack of time is no longer an excuse, as the ten exercises of either course can be practiced in ten minutes if you prefer, although the majority will enjoy training more leisurely than that. Lack of space is no longer an excuse, for this barbell can be used in any space large enough lo stretch the arms to the side, front or overhead. All who have experienced the glad-to-be-alive feeling engendered by barbell training, this new, interesting, and pleasurable way, will never permit themselves to go back to their old slothful form of existing.

Progressive barbell training has long proven to be a superior form of physical training, not only the best way to build strength and muscle, but a means of building internal strength as well. Stronger functional and organic action, stronger hearts, stronger lungs, better acting kidneys, liver, better digestion, superior assimilation, perfect elimination, are the certain and prompt result of progressive barbell training. And experts over all the world, physical training teachers and athletic coaches at famous universities, at schools and colleges, in the army, navy, marine corps, air force and other service groups have pronounced this form of training which is known as Bob Hoffman's Simplified System of Barbell Training, as the very best. They have adopted it in training their men and it has played a most important part in building the fighting men of our nation.

The chief merit of progressive barbell training with a good adjustable barbell, York barbells have long been the leaders, is the fact that it is readily and quickly adaptable to people of every age, both sexes, of every physical condition. In a few seconds the barbell is adjustable from a weight which is suitable for a child, a weak or sick man, an aged man or woman, or a weight which will tax the strength of the strongest, most athletic man. Everyone needs exercise, particularly needs this superior form of training. While most any exorcise is better than no exercise, non-apparatus courses will not bring the results that are desired. You can, regardless of your present age, or physical condition, obtain your physical desires through practicing with this Simplified System of Barbell Training.

The courses to follow are so arranged that every member of the family can use the barbell. Boys and girls, men and women, husbands and wives, sweethearts, groups at the club, at business, should follow Bob Hoffman's Simplified System of Barbell Training. Tell your friends of the splendid results you obtained, how good you feel, they'll see how good you look. The additional members of your family, the man who works next to you at desk or bench, everyone you come into contact with needs this best form of training. Tell them about it so that they can obtain pleasure and physical benefit from it too.

Each Exercise Develops an Important Group of Muscles

WHILE the body contains 720 muscles, these consisting of 4 billion muscular fibres, while they are dosigned lo move the body and its parts in every manner conceivable, making it possible to walk, run, jump, push, pull, lift or carry, while it has been proven through the years that the strongest and best built men, the leaders in the strength world, are those men who have developed and exercised their muscles from every possible angle, the most important muscle groups of the body can be reached and vastly benefited by a comparatively few exercises.

In the first of the streamlined courses offered in this booklet, all the important muscle groups of the body are brought into action, separately. In the second course, the muscle groups are operated in unison, taught to work or coordinate efficiently. The exercises are designed primarily to bring into action all the muscles of the body, particularly the internal muscles and organs. As practically every interna] process is continued in full or in part by muscular action, it's evident that this Course No. 2 is particularly valuable. The heart is a muscle and the huge and powerful American Medical Association backs our long proven theory that the heart strengthens and improves as the result of exercise. Even the lungs, the motivating power of respiration, are largely muscular in their action. The movements of the stomach with resulting improved digestion, better action in the intestines and the bowels, which are entirely muscular in performing their functions, the processes which make you first feel better then look better and be more enduring, are greatly benefited by these movements.

The major muscle groups of the body are: the muscles of the neck, the Trapezius muscles, the muscles on top of the shoulders extending over to the neck, muscles which are the mark of the well-developed, powerful man, and impart the pleasing slope to the shoulders; the Deltoids or muscles of the shoulders; the Biceps, the muscles of the front of the arm; the Triceps, the muscles of the back of the arm; the upper back, the upper chest or Pectoral muscles; the muscles of the sides including the Rhomboids, Serratus Magnus and External Obliques; the muscles which make the back broader, the Latissimus Dorsi group; the vital section, the muscles of the lower back which are so important (they impart strength and vital power to the man, improve his vitality and sexual power); the muscles of the abdomen, which pro- lect and incase the lile sustaining internal organs and processes; the huge muscles of the upper legs, the thighs; the muscles of the call and the complicated muscles of the foot and ankle.

A few minutes spent with either of these two new courses ol Bob Hoffman's Simplified System of Barbell Training will quickly demonstrate to you the muscles which are involved.

The sequence of the exercises requires only seconds in making just two weight changes throughout the movements. The exercises are so arranged that the muscle groups which can handle the least weight are brought into action first. There are three of these exercises consisting of the warm up, the side bend and the two hands curl. Additional weight is added for the fourth exercise, the dead weight lift, the same weight is employed with the two hands press, the rowing motion and the shoulder shrug. Weights are again added and the three heavier and final exercises of the course are practiced.

It is not necessary to reduce the weight of the barbell at any stage, adding weights and changing the "Hold Tite" collars is a matter only of seconds. It's easy for one person to practice these ten body developing exercises in ten minutes. If in a hurry as little as five minutes is required. Four men using the same barbell go through the course without hurrying, taking time to feel the movements every inch of the way, in just twenty minutes.

In Course No. 2 the movements are somewhat similar, but are a bit more advanced. In Course No. 2 there is the usual warm up exercise to get the muscles in action, the blood circulating faster, breathing deeper and more regular. The barbell teetotum instead of the side bend which operates the muscles over a greater range and much more vigorously. Then the back hand curl instead of the front curl which brings into action new individual and groups of muscles. The press behind neck instead of the regular military type of press, which strengthens the arms and shoulders from a new angle. The very vigorous two hands snatch, the "world's best exercise," one which more fully than any other brings into play all the muscles of the outer body, stimulates all the internal works, developing strength, nervous energy, endurance, speed, timing, balance, etc., instead of the much more simple shoulder raise. The "good morning" exercise or bend over instead of the dead weight lift, the upright rowing motion instead of the usual bent over type of rowing motions, with the changed position of the body many different muscles are involved and immensely benefited.

The greatly advanced straddle hop instead of raise on toes, the rapid deep knee bend flat footed instead of the deep knee bend on toes of the first course, and the rapid dead weight lift or cleaning movement instead of the "straddle lift."

All the important muscle groups of the body are brought into definite action in these courses. When you have the time and the inclination, the energy, you could add three special exercises. A neck movement—the neck is the most conspicuous part ol the body when clothed. It is the easiest to develop ol all the muscles, but the first to show signs of age. To be thin and scrawny if you are on the thin side; to be lat, with a long list of double chins, if you are greatly overweight. Your condition is shown to all who observe by your neck, more than any other part. While it receives considerable benefit from nearly all of the movements, the special wrestler's bridge exercise in its various forms will quickly bring the ultimate in neck development, or you can make use of the head or neck strap such as is a part of the

York "Big Twelve Special," the "Seven in One" and the Special "Home Gym," a cable expander set.

Most of the exercises benefit the mid section, particularly all the bending and twisting movements, but you will be benefited even more rapidly if at least once or twice a week you perform a few additional abdominal exercises. The best of these are leg raises while lying, first alone and later with progressive resistance such as with the York Iron Bools. Abdominal raises which can be practiced lying upon a chair with the feet thrust under some heavy immovable object, bending back and touching the head to the floor or sitting up with the inclined abdominal board. The best chest development exercise is the two hands pull over in its various forms. While all the movements ol these courses, particularly those which require more rapid and fuller breathing, will improve the respiration and develop the chest, the two hands pull over will bring most rapid results. This movement is practiced with a barbell of moderate weight, otherwise a good breathing exercise, a chest deepening, expanding movement, will become a muscle developing movement. The weight you employ in the first series should be about right. Lie upon your back on the floor, place barbell at arms' length back of head, keeping the arms straight, pull up overhead and down to the thighs in an arc. Perform the movement slowly and steadily, exhale as the bar goes toward the thighs, inhale very, very deeply as the weight goes back of head. Continue for ten to twenty repetitions. Men with larger, deeper chests are healthiest, and this special exercise, the two hands pull over in its various forms, will bring rapid and superior results.

While it is desirable at times to practice the three suggested added exercises, it is not necessary, for splendid results will be obtained by following the course exactly as it is offered, with ten to fifteen movements in each exercise of the first course and ten different exercises, ten to fifteen repetitions in the second course.

How Exercises Should Be Performed

IT'S a law of life that we get what we pay for in this world. Exercise a little and you obtain favorable results but only in a moderate amount. Exercise more vigorously and greater results are obtained. Vigorous exertion accelerates the action of the vital functions, it creates demands, and nature fills those demands with more strength and muscle, more vital power and endurance.

In handling barbells, certain definite principles should be followed, the most important of which we will endeavor to outline in this little course. There are two ways of holding the barbell. The first known familiarly as the undergrip is seldom used except in the regular two arm curl. With it the bell rests in the palms of the hands as they are raised, palms up and knuckles down. With the overgrip, the one commonly employed in all movements in which the weight is lifted or pulled to the shoulder or overhead, you grasp the bar with the knuckles above the bar and the thumbs below. The usual hand grip is with the hands at shoulder width apart, or approximately 20 inches.

The reverse grip is employed with exercises such as the straddle lift or the heavy dead weight lift. As the name implies, the bar is grasped with the hands in the proper position, shoulder width apart for the dead weight lift, one hand in front of the body, the other to the rear in the straddle lift, and with the palms of the hands facing each other.

The flat back should be employed in all forms of heavy lifting. This prevents soreness of the spine or undue strain of back muscles. In actual weight lifting or heavy deep knee bending the back is always kept flat. In a number of movements such as the stiff legged dead weight lift or the bend over, in which more moderate weights are employed, the back is rounded so that the muscles will receive the greatest range of movement with resulting benefit.

In some of the exercises which you will practice, it is necessary to place the weight upon the shoulders in back of neck. With a fairly heavy weight this is best accomplished by pulling the weight to the chest as in readiness for a regular two arm military press. Then pressing or jerking it over head and lowering it to the back of the neck. With the moderate weight of the usual exercise you can pull the weight up, over and lower it in one continuous movement.

In removing the bell from the shoulders, if it is light enough for you, merely press it to the top of your head, move it forward and lower. If comparatively heavy, give a jump or jerk with the legs to raise it over the head, catch it upon the chest and then lower.

The number of repetitions to employ is most important and is governed chiefly by what you wish to accomplish, and the time and energy you have at your disposal. It is customary to practice most movements from ten to fifteen repetitions. Easier movements such as the shoulder shrug, the raise on toes, the straddle hop. etc., are continued at least until the exercise makes itself felt, certainly more than ten to fifteen movements. In building strength in muscles, tendons and ligaments heavier weights with fewer movements are practiced; for muscle building, ten to fifteen movements are best, and for endurance, higher repetitions are in order. But for the best all around benefit from this course, the usual exercise should be practiced from ten to fifteen movements.

The amount of weight you should use must be determined after consideration of your age, size and weight, present strength and condition, physical desires and ambitions. The courses included in this booklet are primarily designed as get fit and keep fit courses. The really ambitious man, who will wish to go farther by acquiring and training with more weight and more appliances, will train in a somewhat different manner than the man who wishes to keep fit in the easiest possible way. It is best to handle an amount of weight which you can utilize comparatively easily in the beginning. You may be out of condition, or even if in condition the courses of exercises will probably bring into action some little used or seldom used muscles. Slight stiffness or muscular soreness may result. This can be avoided to a great extent by a moderate beginning. But in any event don't be alarmed at the muscular stiffness, it will vanish in a day or two, probably never to return again. I usually say, "make haste slowly," take your time in the beginning. But you must keep in mind as you advance that we pay for what we get in this world and if you wish superior results, you must pay for them with a bit more vigorous work. You will obtain from exercise exactly what you put into it. Take it easy and you will benefit but in a lesser way. Work harder and you will gain more. Less time and energy is required by using fairly heavy weights than light weights, superior results are obtained. So as soon as your muscles are accustomed to the exercise, move up to handling the weight that you can properly use in each exercise the desired number of times without undue strain or fatigue.

In all movements it is desirable that you breathe fully and freely. Therefore it will be necessary during and after the more vigorous exercises that you breathe through the mouth as well as the nose. It is customary in weight training to inhale during the exertion of the movement, and to exhale as the weight or body is lowered. For instance, in two hands pressing, inhale as the weight goes up, exhale as it is lowered to the shoulders. In the deep knee bend inhale as you rise with the weight, exhale as you lower into the full squat position. But this is not absolutely essential, the important matter is to breathe fully enough that the working muscles will be supplied with the oxygen they require so that they can continue with the practice of the repetitions.

When to increase the weight you are using is the next question. There are few men and boys over 16 years of age who will not be able to start with thirty pounds in the first or warm up exercise, continuing this weight in the curl and the side bend. If, due to long neglect of the body or past illnesses, thirty pounds is too heavy, use less weight, the bar alone or the bar with two of the smallest weights placed upon the end. Continue with this weight until it is easy for you to practice fifteen movements. When this point is reached add more weight, an amount that you can conveniently handle for ten repetitions. As your strength increases work up to fifteen again, then add to the weight, reducing the movements to ten. With this system you will eventually reach the point where you can not progress further. Then be satisfied with the weight that you can handle ten to fifteen repetitions, preferably not less than twelve at any time.

Make it a habit to read the descriptions of each exercise thoroughly and often. Until you are far advanced, best to read the description of the exercises each training period. It is highly important that they be followed properly. Otherwise a good arm exercise may become a poor arm and body exercise. There are frequently three or four apparently small details that must be understood and followed. Read the instructions carefully, for your success depends upon the proper execution of each exercise.

Perform all exercises until you are comfortably tired, not exhausted. While it is beneficial, after you are advanced, to work very hard one day a week, you shouldn't work on your nerve too often. The weight you select in each movement should be just enough to make it possible for you to perform the exercises the desired number of times, the number of exercises just enough to leave you comfortably tired at the completion of your training period. You should experience a feeling of exhilaration after you have had your shower or bath and rested a bit.

Some days you will have less pep and energy than others. Don't confuse this lack of pep with laziness. But if you find yourself unable to perform an exercise the expected number of times, let your condition that day be your guide and perform the exercise fewer repetitions. You must be your own instructor to a great extent. For only you know how you feel during and after your training.

With this system of training you should feel better after the first two or three exercise periods. You should then experience a buoyant feeling of well being after your exercise, unless you were too badly out of condition to start. In five to six weeks you should detect noticeable physical improvement. In three months, 13 weeks, at least 52 training periods, you should have made a moderate transformation in your body, inside and out.

When and How to Train

IT is a proven fact that even irregular training with light or moderate weights will benefit you tremendously, provide you with a fair degree of strength, health and development, yet you will accomplish more and get there faster if you follow the simple rules I am about to offer. The courses included in this book, if followed regularly and persistently, will build your body, your muscles and every desirable physical quality in less time and with less effort than with any other system of training.

Persistence is very important. Try not to miss an exercise period. If you do, make up for it by training two days in succession. When you make it a habit of omitting your training you are likely to miss altogether and of course will not obtain beneficial results from the equipment and training instruction you have at your disposal. The longer you continue without missing your training, the surer you are to succeed, for then your training becomes a habit which you will look forward to with pleasurable anticipation.

The ideal way to exercise is every other day, seven times in two weeks. A day of work, a day of rest from exercise, during which nature does its work, meets the demands that have been made upon the body and provides a surplus of strength, energy and endurance. If every other day is not convenient, you could train four or five times a week. With the four times a week system Monday, Wednesday, Thursday and Saturday could be your training days; or Monday, Tuesday, Thursday and Friday. With five times a week: Monday, Tuesday, Wednesday, Thursday and Saturday, or any similar program that suits you will serve well. Be sure however to have two or three days a week during which you do not exercise with your weights or indulge in other forms of athletics. You need these rest days to permit nature to build up your body.

The evening is the best time to exercise, after your day's work is done. Morning exercise brings the organs and muscles into action before they are thoroughly awake, it takes the edge off the day's pep and energy which can better be spent at your profession or vocation. Exercising so that you will have from a half hour to an hour of time before the evening meal, or in the early evening two hours after your evening meal, or so that you will complete your training a half hour or an hour before permanently retiring, are the best times for exercise.

You can spend more time with your training slot if you desire; but you can practice the first course without hurrying in ten minutes. If you have the time and the inclination, remembering that the more you put into exercise the more you get out of it. you can go through both of the courses in one day, or practice other movements which may suggest themselves to you. But be sure to include in each training day's endeavor at least one of the courses exactly as offered in this book. If you become really ambitious and enthused as you probably will, after you experience the splendid results which are the usual effect of exercise, you will desire to obtain more weight. 20 pound weights, 25 pounders, or even 50s and 75s can be obtained to increase the resistance the barbell will offer. Building the ability to handle more weight brings superior results. But rest assured that you will benefit tremendously if you never use a pound more weight than you obtain with the set of weights which accompanies this course.

It is not possible in so brief a course to tell you much about the rules of health. If you make it a habit to read Strength and Health Magazine or obtain some of my books which are devoted to specialized strength and health subjects, you will have all the information about any phase of training you could desire. What should you eat? If you are an overfed business man, wish to regain your normal youthful figure, cut down a bit on what you habitually consume. Eat less of sugars, fats, starches, pastries and other sweets. The underweight person, usually the younger man, needs plenty of good wholesome food to build his body and to replace what he has used up through exercise, and to provide nature with a reserve with which to build more strength and muscle. Eat a variety of good food at meal times only. Beef, mutton, poultry and fish, plenty of leafy vegetables as well as the heavier vegetables and thick soups. For dessert, fruits in various forms, fruit pie, ice cream, custards, etc., will help you build strength and muscle. Weight training men have splendid appetites and can digest most anything. It is only important that the advanced weight man supply his body with ample quantities of all the materials it can require for maintenance and building.

It is my desire to aid you in building your strength and physical powers, but I will make no suggestions which will at any time cause you discomfort. For instance in bathing, use water hardly above the body temperature, never very cold or very hot. Extremely cold water has a shocking effect and it is comfortable to very few. A really hot tub bath is weakening. It will help you sleep better, which is proof that it does weaken you, creating a need and desire for sleep.

Keep yourself warm when training. Well covered. Sun bathing is great, highly beneficial, but it is better to practice sun bathing when not exercising. Particularly during the cooler weather, keep yourself well covered as you go through your training schedule. Perspiration is very beneficial to you.

Don't sleep in a very cold room. This requires energy, as the body must produce a great deal more heat. Sleep where it is comfortable. Seven or eight hours of sleep is the desired amount for most adults. Eight to ten hours is essential for growing boys who are putting forth added effort in following this course of training.

How Much Weight You Should Use

TIME will be saved if the bar is loaded with the smallest plates inside. The 1¼ against the collar, next the 2½, then the 5, the 10 and finally the 12½. This system of loading has several advantages. With the pair of 1¼ weights, the outfit weighs 15; with the 2½ added the weight is 20; with the 5s, 30; with the addition of the pair of 10s, 50; and with the first pair of 12½, the total weight is 75. With this system, the weakest man or woman can use the bar. A small woman or weak man could start with 15 or 20 pounds, an average man with 30 pounds in the first exercise. A man a bit farther advanced could easily perform the first series of three exercises with 50 pounds, or even 75.

While this course was originally designed to be used with the York Aristocrat Barbell, the weights of which are as indicated above, it also serves well with the Victory and War Time York Barbells. The steel pipe bar of the Victory set weighs 7½ pounds, with the 1¼ pound plates you have an even 10 pounds to start with. With the War Time, the painted steel bar weighs 15 pounds; the 20. 30, 50 of the Aristocrat weights in the first series are possible with the War Time, but in the second series, instead of 30, 50, 75, you can have 30, 45, 75 with all iron plates up to 45 and then a pair of Composition plates and in the third series the 50, 75, 100 of the Aristocrat will be 45, 75, 100 or 105.

When several people are to exercise with one barbell, time will be saved if persons of nearly equal strength will use the same barbell. In training of service groups of the Army, Navy, Marine Corps, Air Force, Sea Bees and Merchant Marine, with groups of C. C. C. camps, at boys' camps, at school, Y. M. C. A.'s, this new barbell and simplified system of barbell training offers a means of building strength and muscle, a good basis for athletics, work and the general business of living. Four men should have no difficulty in performing all the exercises of one course in twenty minutes, performing the exercises without undue haste so that the most beneficial results can be had by feeling the weight resistance every inch of the way as the weight is raised and lowered.

If you were training a group of men or women and desired to have your charges work in at least a semi-military fashion, which of course is the best way for large groups to exercise, you would have groups of four men with each barbell. The smallest man should be first in line, the others stand in line back of him at ease with hands on hips or clasped in rear of back, feet a comfortable distance apart. Using a system of exercising by the counts, after the first man has taken his position in front of the barbell, the instructor would give the command. Ready. Then the count, one-two, at the count of one bend over and grasp the bell, at the count of two stand up with the weight at the starting position. After a slight pause, the command, Ready-Exercise. The movements start with the count one-two-three-four, one-two-three-four, then up-down or down-up depending upon the exercise, to illustrate that it is the fifth repetition; then one-two-three-four, one-two- three-four, then up-halt.

As each man completed his movements he would face to the right, take two strides, face to the right again and take his place at the rear of the line. In a comparatively short time, each of the four men using the barbell will complete the first three exercises, the warm up, the side bend and the regular curl. The last man to use the barbell and the man next in line take their places to add to the weight, and with the Hold Tite collars and the addition of two plates, the 10s for men who have started with 30, the 12½ for men who have started with 50, the weight is increased to the desired amount.

The same procedure is followed with the dead lift, the press, the shoulder shrug and the rowing motion. The change is made again, adding another pair of 12'/ss for advanced men, bringing the weight to 100 pounds in all; and the remaining three exercises have their turn. The raise on toes, straddle lift and deep knee bend on toes. The second course is more vigorous but requires even less time as the exercises are performed more rapidly. A similar procedure is employed in practicing these ten exercises.

One of the best ways to perform this simplified course of barbell training is to employ the system of compound exercises. By this I mean performing the first three exercises in succession without setting the weight down. This is not too difficult as different muscles are involved in each movement. At the same time better results are obtained because one must work harder, breathe harder, blood circulates faster, perspiration is induced, one completes the series of three, breathing faster, heart beating more rapidly and forcefully and of course good results are obtained from these more vigorous exercises. A man must be strong to complete the middle series of four exercises without stopping, but if he can do it, good results are obtained. If four exercises are too difficult, complete two in succession. Rest a moment, or if training with a group wait until others have had their turn, then perform the other two. It is not difficult to perform the last three exercises in series as a compound movement, for the weight rests on the shoulders in two of the exercises, the muscles involved are the largest and strongest in the body so unusual fatigue will not be experienced.

With this compound system of training I have performed the entire series of ten exercises, 12 repetitions each, starting with 50 in the first series, advancing to 75 in the second and 100 in the third, in just 5 minutes. With 15 repetitions, at least seven minutes are required. It is seldom necessary to hurry so fast, but when time is short I have done it. The normal procedure in following this simplified system of training is to take your time, rest well between movements. Good results will be obtained with a minimum of exertion or fatigue.

In training with a family group or any group made up of persons of greatly diversified strength, time is saved if each of the group will complete one series before changing the weight. For instance, the group may consist of father, mother and young son. Mother is in fairly good muscular condition as she has been taking part in the exercises for some time. She can employ 30 pounds in the first series. Young son is becoming pretty husky so he can use 50, and father, a barbell man of considerable experience, will perform the first series with 75. Each performs their three exercises either as a compound series or with a short rest between. In the second series, 50 pounds for mother, 75 for the young son, 100 for father. In the third series 75 pounds for mother, 100 for the son and 125 for father who has procured some additional weights so he can obtain more from his exercises. If mother were not as strong nor as ambitious, she could start with 20 in series 1, 30 in series 2 and 50 in the last series.

Husbands and wives, young men and women, sweethearts or at least training pals, groups of young men at home or at the club, during an outing at the beach, mountain, or stream, or larger groups will find this simplified system of barbell training easily adaptable to their needs.

My last and perhaps most important bit of advice is to do what you should before you do what you like. Barbell training is so fascinating; there are many lifts and strength feats which can be practised. There is so much temptation to deviate from the course and try oneself out or have competition with other members of a group before the exercises of one of the courses are completed. But make it a rule from which you never deviate, that you go through one complete series of ten movements, either of the first or second courses, before you permit yourself to do anything else. When you have done what you should, practiced one of the regular body building courses, which bring into action all the major muscle groups of the body, then you can do what you like. Physical training is like putting money in the bank. Save regularly little by little and over a considerable period you will have a fair bank account. But save just as regularly and a little more each week and your bank account will grow just as surely and much more rapidly. Similarly, exercise a little and regularly and you will greatly improve your physical condition. But train a little harder, train just as regularly and soon your strength and health bank account will make you a very rich person physically. Make it possible for you to obtain the fullest measure of health, strength, happiness and success from life. Good luck to you.

How to Use the Courses

THE ten exercises of the 1st course of the Simplified Barbell Training System in proper sequence and grouped according to weight increases are:

1.   TWO HANDS HIGH PULL UP

2.   SIDE TO SIDE BEND

3.   TWO HANDS REGULAR CURL

(Weight increase of 50%)

4.   STIFF LEG DEAD LIFT

5.   TWO HANDS MILITARY PRESS

6.   SHOULDER SHRUG

7.   ROWING MOTION

(Weight increase of 50%)

8.   RAISE ON TOES

9.   STRADDLE LIFT

10.   REGULAR DEEP KNEE BEND

On the following pages each exercise is clearly described. The parts of the body developed by each exercise are given, after which follows the amount of weight used. The description of performance of the movement is given in bold type, each separate motion is identified by three dots. The diagram at the side of each description shows the starting and finishing position and each of these positions is numbered and referred to in the description as (Position No. 1, Position No. 2, etc.). The numbers of repetitions are then given. After each description, in lighter type, are some notes of correct procedure.

READ ALL THESE CAREFULLY AND BECOME COMPLETELY FAMILIAR WITH ENTIRE TEXT.

TWO HANDS HIGH PULL-UP

Warming up exercise

NOTE: Select starting weight in manner described in text.

Stand close to barbell, foot 12 to 18 inches apart ... grasp barbell with both hands a bit more than shoulder width apart (Position No. 1 in diagram) ... straighten up pulling barbell to a point a few inches above the head (Position No. 2 in diagram) ... lower the weight stopping barbell as it almost touches the floor (Position No. 3 in diagram) ... continue

movement (Position No. 1) ... do from 10 to 15 repetitions.

Use a weight light enough that you can pull up as described. At completion of upward movement (Position No. 2) arms should be overhead and legs straight. This is not a strength feat but merely a warming up exercise. The movement should be done slowly enough that exertion can be felt every inch of the way. There is no pause during any part of this movement.

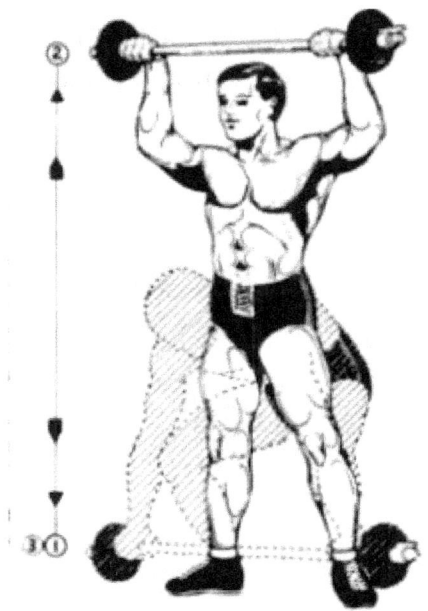

SIDE TO SIDE BEND

Develops all the muscles of the sides

Stand close to bar - feet 12 to 18 inches apart ... grasp barbell with both hands at full width ... lift to chest ... from chest lift overhead and place on back of neck (Position No. 1) ... bend slowly and steadily as far to the left as possible (Position No. 2) ... pause for two seconds ... bend as far to the right as possible ... (Position No. 3) ... pause ... repeat movement ... do 20 repetitions (10 left and 10 right).

Keep legs straight at all times. Bend only to side, do not allow trunk to bend forward. Breathe deeply.

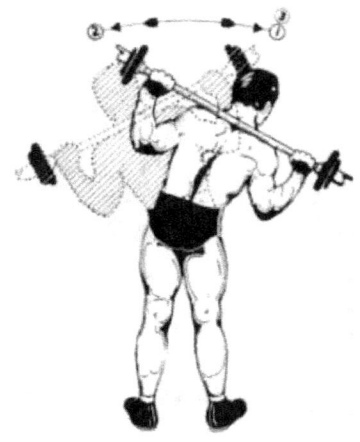

TWO HANDS REGULAR CURL

Develops muscles of arm.

Stand close to barbell ... grasp barbell with both hands, PALMS OUT ... stand erect (Position No. 1) ... slowly, without moving elbows, curl weight to shoulders (Position No. 2) ... lower barbell to first position (Position No. 3) ... continue movement ... do from 10 to 15 repetitions.

Exercise must be done slowly with strength of arms alone. Do not lean backward. Keep elbows close to sides with as little movement as possible. Breathe deeply.

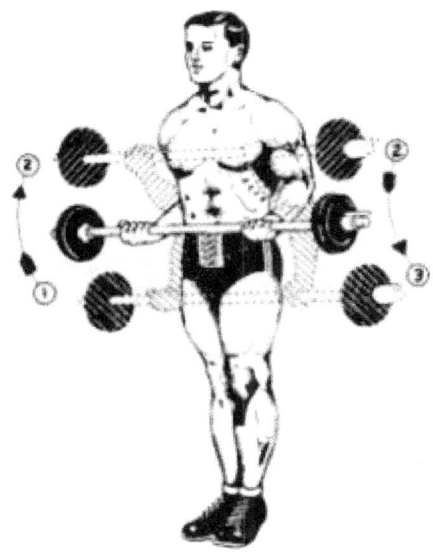

STIFF LEG DEAD LIFT

Develops powerful muscles of lower back

NOTE: Increase weight of barbell 50% over exercises 1, 2 and 3.

Stand close to barbell, feet 12 to 18 inches apart ... grasp barbell with both hands at shoulder width ... stand erect, barbell against thighs (Position No. 1) ... without bending legs lower barbell until it nearly touches floor (Position No. 2) ... come back to erect position (Position No. 3) ... continue movement... do 15 repetitions.

Do not bend knees, keep legs straight at all times. Turn toes out slightly for better balance. This exercise gives you extreme flexibility. As you progress you can perform movements on a box permitting barbell to go lower than feet.

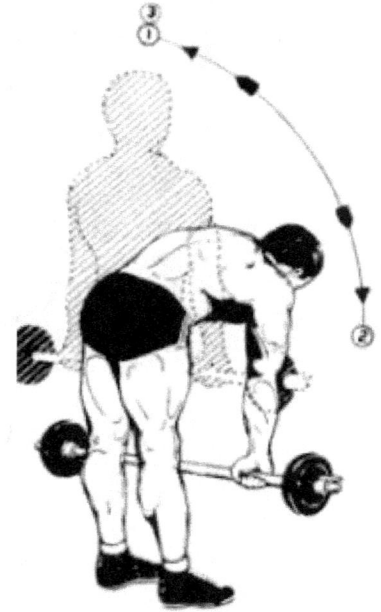

TWO HANDS MILITARY PRESS

Develops shoulders and triceps.

Stand close to barbell, feet 12 to 18 inches apart ... grasp barbell with both hands at shoulder width ... lift to chest (Position No. 1) ... Steadily push barbell to arm's length overhead (Position No. 2) ... lower to chest (Position No. 3) and repeat movement ... do 10 to 15 repetitions.

Keep legs straight, back should not bend during this movement. Do not look up at the barbell but keep eyes to front. Resist the weight when lowering it to the chest. Breathe deeply.

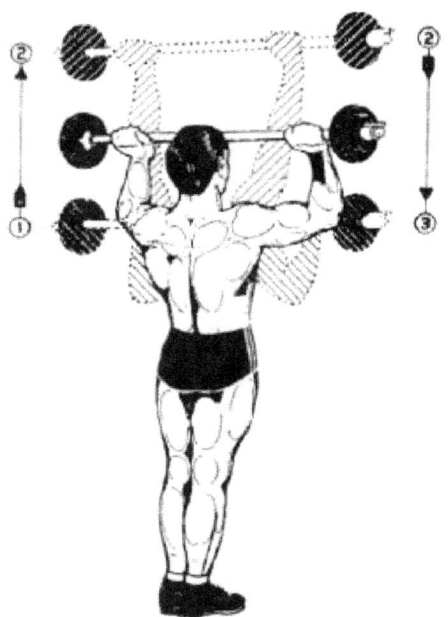

SHOULDER SHRUG

Develops trapezius muscles.

Stand close to barbell, feet 12 to 18 inches apart ... grasp barbell with both hands slightly more than shoulder width apart ... stand erect, barbell against thighs (Position No. 1) ... without bending elbows raise shoulders as high as possible (Position No. 2) ... lower (Position No. 3) ... continue movement ... do 15 to 20 repetitions.

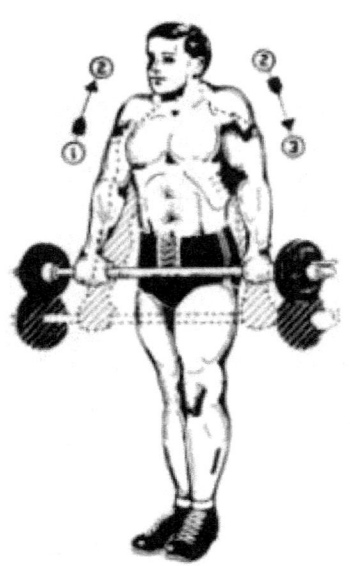

Keep arms straight at all times. Force shoulders as high as you can, pausing at extreme height for a second before lowering. Exhale when lowering.

ROWING MOTION

Develops muscles of upper back and all of upper arm

Stand close to barbell, feet 12 to 18 inches apart ... grasp barbell with both hands slightly more than shoulder width apart ... lift a few inches from the floor without bending legs (Position No. 1) ... with upper body still bent over, pull barbell to chest (Position No. 2) ... lower to within a few inches of floor (Position No. 3) ... continue movement ... do 10 to 15 repetitions.

Lift barbell without raising upper body. Keep legs straight at all times. Keep elbows a bit front as weight touches chest. Lower barbell slowly, resisting weight all the way. Breathe deeply.

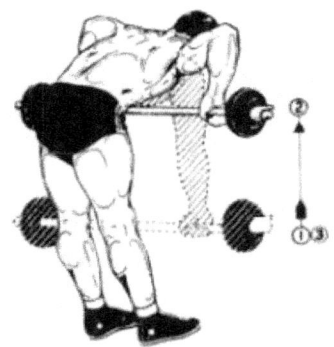

RAISE ON TOES

Develops calves and strengthens feet and arch.

NOTE: Increase weight of barbell 50% over exercises 4, 5, 6, and 7.

Stand close to barbell, feet 12 to 18 inches apart... grasp barbell with both hands at extreme width ... pull barbell up to chest ... lift barbell overhead and place on back of neck (Position No. 1) ... raise up on toes as far as possible (Position No. 2) ... lower heels to floor (Position No. 3) ... continue movement ... do 10 repetitions with feet in each position. 30 repetitions in all.

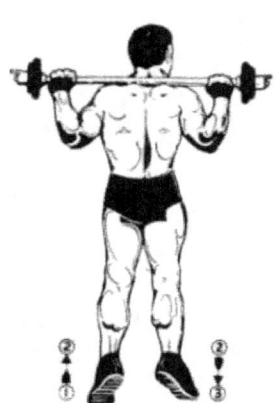

Knees must not be bent. The exercise can be varied by turning toes well out during one period and turned in on other periods and at other times straight to the front.

STRADDLE LIFT

Develops most muscles of upper leg and increases flexibility.

Stand astride the barbell, feet about 18 inches apart ... grasp bar with both hands, one in front of body, one behind (Position No. 1) ... stand erect lifting barbell to crotch (Position No. 2) ... lower almost to floor (Position No. 3) ... continue movements ... do 10 to 15 repetitions.

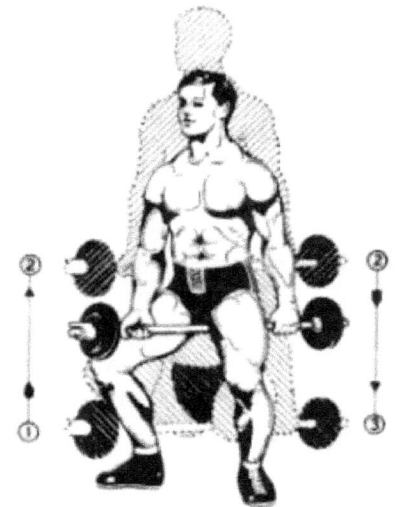

Perform with moderate slowness. Keep back straight. Breathe deeply.

DEEP KNEE BEND ON TOES

Develops all muscles of body and teaches balance.

Stand close to barbell, feet 12 to 18 inches apart ... grasp barbell with both hands slightly more than shoulder width apart ... lift barbell to chest... lift barbell overhead and place 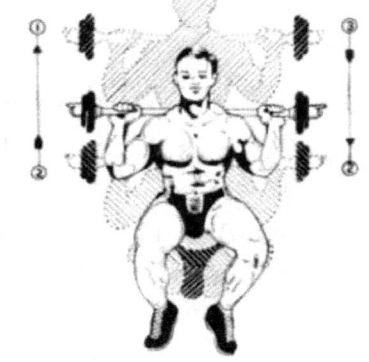 **across back of neck (Position No. 1) ... raise on toes ... lower body into full squat position (Position No. 2) ... come to erect position (Position No. 3) ... repeat movement ... do 10 to 15 repetitions.**

The most difficult part of this exercise is the balancing on toes, but once mastered you have no trouble. Breathe deeply while lowering body into full squat, exhale then inhale again before arising. Later the exercise may be practiced with heels together. Come to the erect position as fast as possible and keep from leaning forward.

Second Course of Bob Hoffman's Simplified System of Barbell Physical Training

WHILE Course No. 1 includes a barbell system of unusual merit, one which brings into favorable action all of the principal muscle groups of the body, Course No. 2 of Bob Hoffman's Simplified System of Barbell Physical Training in many ways is superior, more result producing than the first course. It is intended that this more vigorous course be included in the training of the new barbell man only after at least a month has been spent in conditioning the muscles with the exercises of the first course.

Exercises which involve all the muscles, particularly those of the mid-section, possess unusual merit and bring superior results. In nearly every exercise of this Course No. 2. practically all of the muscles of the body are brought into action. The muscles which have been developed in groups in the first course are now taught to work in unison so that many other desirable physical qualities are produced, in addition to the strength and muscle building which a properly designed system of barbell training will produce if properly and persistently followed. Balance, endurance, speed, judgment of space and distance, improved digestion, assimilation and respiration, as well as better operation of every bodily process is the certain result of following this Course No. 2.

Every barbell man should mentally sign a pledge to include one or both of these training courses in each day's weight training. After you have performed the ten exercises of Course No. 1 or Course No. 2, exercises which will produce a balanced development as well as internal strength and power in the outer muscles, you can do anything else that you like. Too many men in using their barbell set do not follow the regular course, just "tinker" along and therefore receive only mediocre results. Constantly keep in mind that you obtain from barbell work what you put into it, and plan to put enough in it that you will receive results satisfactory to yourself. The merits of barbell training are judged by the results that you as an individual who are training with weights obtain, and if you do not train properly and live wisely, thus obtaining superior results, you do harm to the best system of physical training. If you enjoy including weight lifting, tumbling or hand balancing in your program, if you like to wrestle and box or play hand ball, take a swim or just play some game, if you like to specialize on the exercises at which you are best, to devote most of your training time to the exercises at which you excel, that's your privilege.

But determine, please, to perform the exercises you should before you go on to do what you prefer to do. The inclusion of one of these complete courses in every day's training will guarantee your success, guarantee that your body will be strong all over, inside and out, that you will have a symmetrical development If you train at home or at a club where weights are the chief medium of training, don't fail to practice one of these complete simplified courses, urge all other members of your club, your group, your friends and acquaintances to practice one of these complete training courses, each training day. Every barbell man is judged by the results he obtains, help the barbell movement, help others as well as yourself by never failing to practice one of these complete courses in conjunction with other exercises you may wish to do on your regular training day.

THE ten exercises of the Second or Advanced Course of the Simplified Barbell

Training System in proper sequence and grouped according to weight increases are:

1.   TWO HANDS PRESS COMPLETE

2.   TWO HANDS REVERSE CURL

3.   BARBELL TEETOTUM

(Weight increase of 50%)

4.   PRESS FROM BEHIND NECK

5.   TWO   HANDS   REPETITION SNATCH

6.   BARBELL BEND OVER

7.   UPRIGHT ROWING MOTION

(Weight increase of 50%)

8.   REGULAR DEEP KNEE BEND

9.   BARBELL STRADDLE HOP

10.   RAPID HIGH DEAD LIFT

NOTE: Select starting weight in manner described in text.

TWO HANDS PRESS COMPLETE

Warming up exercise

Stand close to barbell, feet 12 to 18 inches apart ... grasp barbell with both hands about shoulder width apart (Position No. 1) ... lift barbell to chest (Position No. 2) ... press barbell to arm's length overhead (Position No. 3) ... lower barbell to chest (Position No. 4) ... lower barbell from chest to floor (Position No. 5) ... continue movements ... do 10 to 15 repetitions.

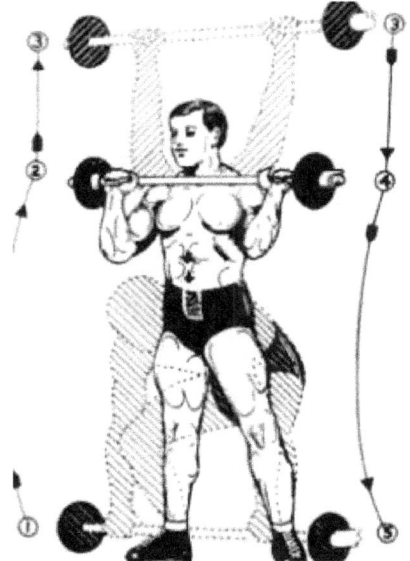

This movement should be performed so that the weight is felt every inch of the way. The back should be kept straight as possible, while pressing the barbell from the chest to arm's length overhead. Breathe deeply at all times.

Although this movement is here suggested as a warm up exercise, it is one of the very best exercises in physical training, a great many body builders consider it the very best, it should have a more important part in your training. Advanced barbell men frequently perform Exorcise No. 5, of course No. 1, the Two Hands Military Press, or Exercise 4 of Course No. 2, in this continuous pull-up and press style. In this latter case the weight is pulled up and in back of head in one continuous movement. It takes a pretty good man to perform 15 repetitions with 100 pounds in this style. If you have so little time some day that you consider seriously missing your training for that day, perform this continuous pull-up and press, and the deep knee bend. Hardly more than two or three minutes will be required and you will receive a good share of benefit from this abbreviated training program.

TWO HANDS REVERSE CURL

Develops muscles of the forearm and bicep.

Stand close to barbell, feet 12 to 18 inches apart ... grasp barbell with both hands' palms facing in, about shoulder width apart ... stand erect bringing barbell to thighs (Position No. 1) ... curl barbell to shoulders (Position No. 2) ... lower barbell to thighs (Position No. 3) ... repeat movement ... do 10 to 15 repetitions.

It is important that the elbows be held at the sides, and that there is no swinging of the body to assist in performing the movement. The exercise should be performed slowly, so the weight can be felt the entire way.

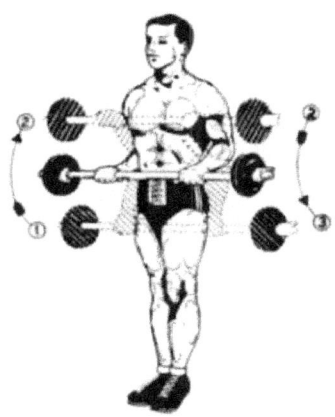

BARBELL TEETOTUM

Develops muscles of the side and also the back.

Stand close to bar, feet 18 to 24 inches apart ... grasp the bar with both hands slightly more than shoulder width apart ... stand erect bringing barbell to thighs (Position No. 1) ... swing trunk at the same time bending to the right, touching barbell to the floor (Position No. 2) ... (right knee is bent slightly) ... come to erect position (Position No. 1) ... swinging trunk at the same time bending to the left touching barbell to the floor (Position No. 3) ... (left knee is bent slightly) ... come to erect position (Position No. 1) ... repeat movements ... do 10 to 15 repetitions.

It is one of the best side exercises and it also involves with beneficial effect all the muscles of the back.

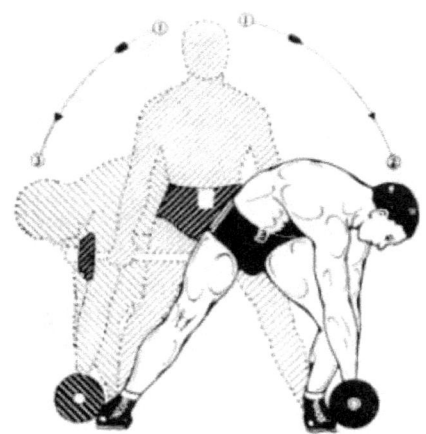

PRESS FROM BEHIND NECK

Develops the shoulders and arms

NOTE: Increase weight of barbell 50% over exercises 1, 2 and 3.

Stand close to barbell, feet 12 to 18 inches apart ... grasp the bar with both hands slightly more than shoulder width apart ... lift barbell to chest ... lift overhead and place on neck (Position No. 1) ... press to arm's length overhead (Position No. 2) ... lower to back of neck (Position No. 3) ... repeat movement ... do 10 to 15 repetitions.

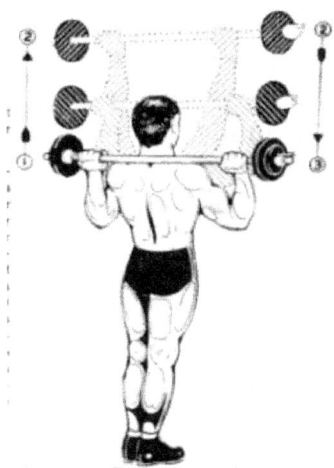

Do not fail to touch the back of the nock with the barbell, after each repetition. This exercise involves the entire shoulder assembly and particularly develops the muscles of the arms and shoulders. It brings the muscles into action in a somewhat different manner than in the two hands press of Course No. 1, with resulting beneficial developmental effect.

TWO HANDS REPETITION SNATCH

Develops all muscles of the body and builds stamina.

Stand close to bar, feet 12 to 18 inches apart ... grasp barbell with both hands at extreme width (Position No. 1) ... with one long and continuous pull lift barbell from floor to arm's length overhead, at the same time moving one foot forward and one foot backwards (Position No. 2) ... bring feet together, front foot first then back foot, thus stand erect with barbell overhead (Position No. 3) ... lower barbell from arm's length overhead to within a few inches of the floor and repeat movement ... do 10 to 15 repetitions.

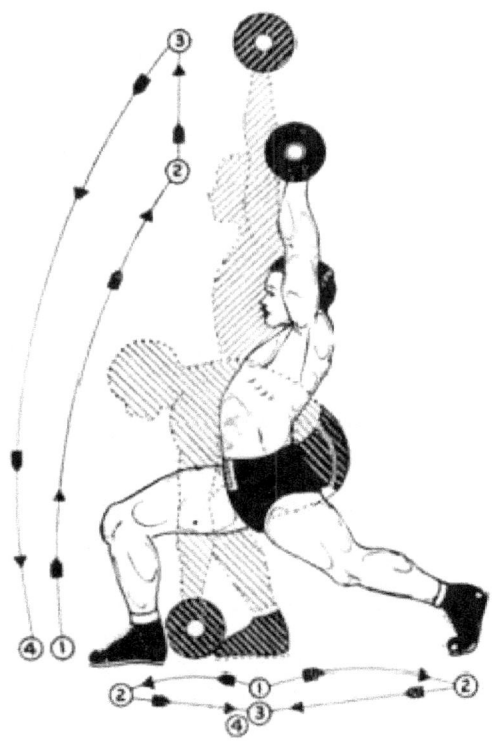

This is the best single exercise in the entire line of physical training. When lifting barbell to arm's length overhead KEEP THE BAR CLOSE TO THE BODY. The upward movement of the barbell should be vigorous and as fast as possible. The feet should be split fore and aft as fast as physically possible just as the bar reaches the chin. The arms shoot out overhead as the feet touch the floor

(Position No. 2). The feet leave the ground at the same time and should touch the floor at the completion of the split at the same time, NOT ONE AFTER THE OTHER. The forward leg is bent and the backward leg is kept straight (as shown in Position No. 2). The legs are brought together, however, alternately, first the front then the back leg.

Before starting this exercise, determine which way it is easier to split. Most bodybuilders find it easier to move the left leg forward and the right leg backward, but determine for yourself which suits.

BARBELL BEND-OVER

Develops lumbar region of lower back

Stand close to barbell, feet 12 to 18 inches apart ... grasp barbell with both hands slightly more than shoulder width apart ... lift barbell to chest... lift barbell from chest overhead and place on back of neck (Position No. 1) ... without bending knees, lean forward as far as possible (Position No. 2) ... come to erect position (Position No. 3) ... repeat movement ... do 10 to 15 repetitions.

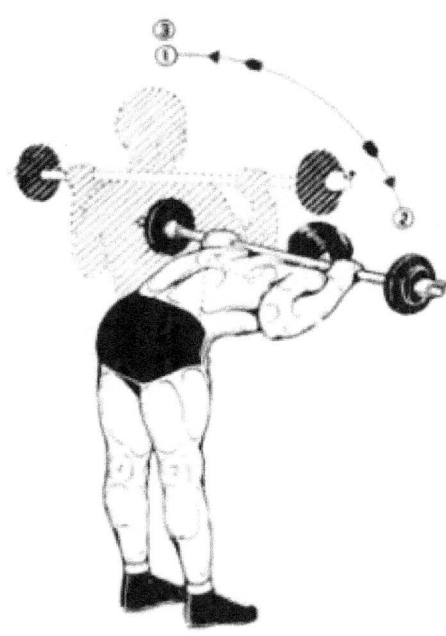

It is important to keep the legs straight. As you practice you will be able to bend much farther forward.

Besides strengthening the lower back, this movement also builds the back of the upper legs and massages the internal organs.

UPRIGHT ROWING MOTION

Develops upper arms, trapezius and back of shoulders.

Stand close to barbell, feet 12 to 18 inches apart ... grasp barbell with hands shoulder width apart ... straighten legs, lifting

barbell from floor to thighs (Position No. 1) ... while still standing erect draw barbell up to chin (Position No. 2) ... lower barbell to starting position at thighs (Position No. 3) ... repeat movement ... do 10 to 15 repetitions.

Keep the legs straight and move the upper body as little as possible, drawing bar to chest by arm strength alone. This exercise gives splendid bulk to the upper arm. Breathe deeply while lifting barbell.

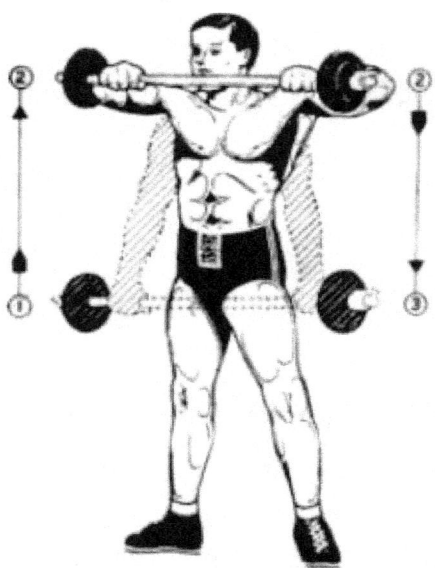

REGULAR DEEP KNEE BEND

Develops nearly all muscles of body, back and thighs while enforced breathing enlarges chest

Note: Increase weight of barbell 50% over exercises 4, 5, 6 and 7.

Stand close to barbell, feet 12 to 18 inches apart ... grasp barbell with both hands slightly more than shoulder width apart ... pull barbell up to chest ... lift barbell overhead and place on back of neck (Position No. 1)... lower yourself into full squat position (Position No. 2) ... come up to erect position (Position No. 3) do 15 repetitions.

Deep breathing is an important part of this exercise which is one of the best body building movements known. Inhale deeply at the start, exhale while lowering into full squat position and again inhale deeply while arising. Keep the back as straight as possible and avoid leaning forward as much as possible.

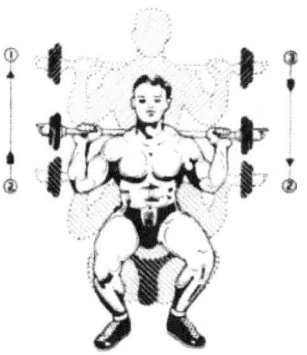

BARBELL STRADDLE HOP

Develops thighs, calves, strengthens feet and imparts springiness to legs.

Stand close to barbell, feet together ... grasp barbell with both hands slightly more than shoulder width apart ... lift barbell to chest ... lift barbell from chest overhead and place across back of neck (Position No. 1) ... jump, spreading the legs apart sideways (Position No. 2) without pausing jump, bringing feet together again (Position No. 3) and without pausing repeat movement ... do 15 to 20 repetitions.

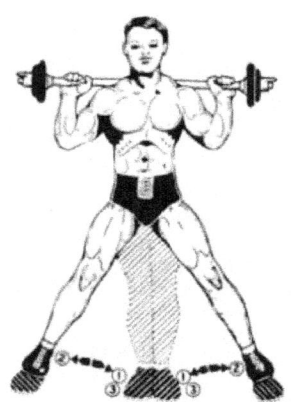

This is a jumping or springing movement and there should be no pause during the entire drill. Hold bar tightly against neck, or somewhat lower for more comfort, and do not let it bounce against neck. Later you can vary this exercise by alternately splitting the feet fore and aft. Breathe deeply throughout entire drill.

RAPID HIGH DEAD LIFT

Develops all upper body muscles

Stand close to barbell, feet 12 to 18 inches apart ... grasp bar with both hands shoulder width apart (Position No. 1) ... with one quick continuous movement lift barbell from floor to a point even with nipples (Position No. 2) and without pausing, lower barbell to within a few inches of floor (Position No. 3) ... and without pausing repeat movement ... do 10 to 15 repetitions.

This exercise, often called the cleaning movement, builds terrific strength into the upper body. It develops the small of the back and improves posture. Speed and a continuous movement are required throughout this drill. Keep the elbows high. Breathe deeply at all times.

Many body builders for variation like to use a much narrower grip and practice pulling up to chin in this movement. With this style it brings the muscles into action in a somewhat different manner. This is one of the very best exercises in the entire line of physical training. Physical directors of the Royal Canadian Air Force, who use this Simplified system, urge their men to practice at least three movements, continuous pull up and press, deep knee bend and high pull up or rapid dead weight lift.

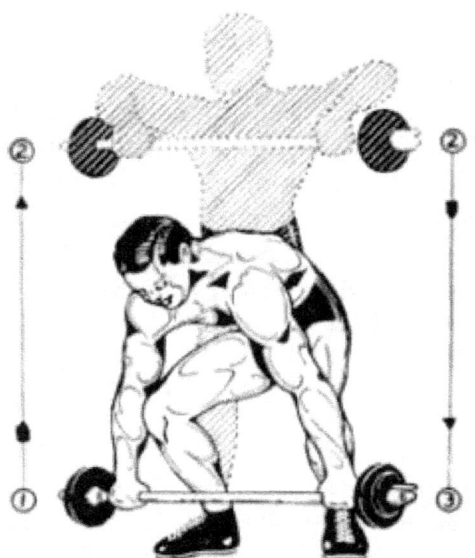

I AM sure that after you have practiced this series of movements for a time you will be enthused at the way you feel and pleased to see the great improvement in your physical appearance. While I have asked you to include one of these courses in each day's training, when you have time and are particularly energetic, performing the entire twenty movements is not too much. I have made it a habit to practice one or both of these courses after practicing weight lifting with our team, and it sends me away from the gym feeling like a million. It is nice too to use the set of weights which we have ready for action in our music room.

With such fine courses so simply and scientifically arranged no one has a legitimate excuse not to taste the multitude of benefits which are the direct result of a proper course in weight training. While most of the exercises in this course are generally known, the manner in which they are arranged, the copyrighted sequence and description of the exercises, guarantees the beneficial results. They are arranged in a unique time-saving manner. You're sure to obtain splendid results if you persist. Good luck to you.

Normalize Your Weight

ACCORDING to statistics in the United States there are 37 million underweight adults, eighteen million overweight adults. Aside from the 37 million underweight adults there are a great many young men and women, not yet mature or developed, who desire to increase their bodyweight. Those who seek to gain weight with bar bell training undoubtedly outweigh those who seek to reduce their weight, by at least two to one. You who read this may be in one category or the other, so this course would not be complete without offering you advice and information concerning the best way to normalize your body, gain weight if underweight, lose weight if overweight at present.

First you should endeavor to attain the bodyweight which is normal for your height and bony framework. When deciding if your weight is normal, after consulting the chart of height and weight, be fair with yourself. Although your weight may apparently check with the correct poundage for your age, height and skeletal construction, if you have thin arms and legs and a too generous waist line, your mirror will tell you that you need to reduce your waist and build the size and strength of your limbs. An overweight condition is not only unsightly, not only a sign of ignorance, gluttony or laziness but is positively dangerous as well. Carrying pounds of weighty unsightly fat burdens your organs, and greatly restricts their action.

By taking an inventory of your physical self you will be in a position to place yourself in the category to which you belong, the moderately overweight, the pleasingly plump, the greatly overweight, the definitely fat, a bit underweight or greatly emaciated. If you are normal in weight, your body normalizing task is easy, for then you need only build your strength and to supply your body with foods to maintain your body at the peak physically. If you are overweight you must make it a habit to consume foods which will not add to your weight. You shouldn't entirely dispense with fats such as butter, nut meats or animal proteins, even if you are overweight, but you should know, when you are overweight, that to normalize your body you must reduce the quantity of fat producing foods you consume and to exercise more.

If you are underweight, you need more of the body and weight building foods. Whether overweight or underweight your success will result in great measure according to your knowledge of foods and their properties. While the barest essentials only can be included in a course of this size, you will guarantee your success by obtaining more complete information on physical training and right living such as is contained in some of my books, notably Better Nutrition, a complete treatise on foods, and their properties, minerals and vitamins. How to Be Strong, Healthy and Happy and the specialized books such as Secrets of Strength and Development, Big Arms, the Big Chest Book, Weight Lifting, etc. By having a more complete knowledge of foods it will greatly assist you in gaining or losing weight, and you will be sure to supply your body with every one of the 16 mineral elements it requires. Set a goal for yourself to lose twenty pounds, to gain twenty pounds, depending upon your bodyweight at present. As the majority are underweight you will no doubt desire to add pounds of good solid, powerful muscle to your frame. You may have some annoying ailment to overcome. At any rate, it will be much easier for you to keep your goal constantly before you if you write down what you intend to accomplish. Thus you can constantly have before you your ambitions, aims and desires, as you visualize the task you have set for yourself.

Just remember please, whether you wish to gain weight or lose weight, the most important means to that end is the selection of the foods you should eat. For to obtain quick and satisfying results from your physical endeavors, you must live right, coordinate your eating properly and exercise properly and persistently. Before going on with correct eating, one of the most important essentials of health, I wish to impart a few words about correct living.

I constantly list the four main essentials of health as correct eating, proper sleep and relaxation, the maintenance of a tranquil mind and the right sort of exercise. There is considerable in this course concerning exercise. I intend to supply the essentials of eating. Be certain you obtain sufficient sleep. This leaves the maintenance of a tranquil mind and many minor but nevertheless important phases of living which you should take into consideration. There are a number of reasons for failure to obtain the proper results from your training. Heading the list is not enough of the right kind of exercise, not working hard enough, some few fail by training too hard but these are greatly in the minority. If you follow the other essentials of health you will benefit from large quantities of exercise. The wrong kind of exercise accounts for many failures, but the inability of the body to respond to exercise is also of great importance.

This may delay your progress at first; possibly through inheritance you have less internal organic and glandular strength than normal, perhaps through the life you have led, loss of sleep, too much eating, drinking, smoking, or sexual excesses you have so weakened your body that it will not immediately and fully respond to physical training such as is offered in this course. To speed the progress you obtain you must change your mode of living. Proper living and exercise is a great healer of disease, in short of what ails you; if you have a subnormal beginning it will require a reasonable period to so improve your bodily processes that you obtain the most favorable results from your training.

The practice of moderation in all things is the best advice I can offer you. You will gain best if you give up entirely all harmful habits. If this is too difficult for you, at least cut them to a bare minimum. These habits will include smoking, drinking of alcoholic beverages, even of coffee, loss of sleep, sexual excesses, and dissipations of any kind.

While moderate smoking or moderate drinking of stimulating beverages alone will not harm you greatly, it is the combination of all of these things, the adding together of all the leaks, which ultimately weakens your body and greatly retards your physical progress when once you have launched out upon a program of physical betterment.

ONLY with training apparatus which permits graded progress, can you measure your gains, know how you compare this day with last week, last month and last year, and only with the progressive system can you gain steadily and without strain of any sort. With barbells, or their partner, adjustable dumbells, the weakest man or woman, one who is recovering from illness, injuries or battle wounds, one who is badly out of condition, can start with a very light weight, the weight of the bar alone, and from this point, using the progressive system with moderate weight increases, can advance to the point where there is sufficient resistance for the strongest man.

The most generally used method to progress is from 10 to 15 repetitions. However, if you are weak, or badly out of condition, you can start with 5 and the single or double progressive system. Unless you have great handicaps to overcome the single progressive system will normally serve you well. If you are very weak, a wounded veteran for instance, you select a weight which is easy for you to handle 5 repetitions, You rest the next day, and then on the third training day again practice 5 repetitions, rest the 4th, 6 repetitions the 5th, rest the 6th, 6 repetitions the 7th, rest the 8th, 7 repetitions the 9th. rest the 10th, and continue in this way until on the 21st day 10 repetitions are reached.

At this point you must determine what to do, for only you know how you feel and how your muscles and internal system have responded to progressive training. If you are not feeling full of pep, feeling much stronger, increase the weight by only 5 pounds and start again with 5 repetitions working up to 10 as described. Continue to use the double progressive system as you reach ten counts, adding to the weight and again reducing to 5 movements.

But if this three weeks of training has placed you in good condition as it will unless you have a particularly bad start, you can then work from 10 to 15 repetitions using either the double or single progressive system. The average fellow can start with a weight he can handle for ten repetitions; if the double progressive system is used it will require three weeks to go from 10 to 15 repetitions, but if the single progressive system is employed it will take but ten days. Most men will find it best to use the double progressive system from 10 to 15, with either the 20-30-50 series or the 30-50-75 series. As you follow this system for a time, you'll learn that 15 repetitions with 50-75-100, and both courses, provides a very good workout.

The every other day system of training is the simplest, but if you do not wish to train on Sunday, you can arrange your training days so that you exercise three days, Monday, Wednesday and Friday, or if four days, Monday, Wednesday. Thursday. Saturday. If particularly ambitious you could train 5 days, but be sure to have from two to four days a week in which to refrain from special exercise. It is essential in this form of training that you extend yourself at times, and then have days of rest during which the body does its building work so that you attain your physical desires.

Correct Eating is Important

WHILE it is true that some strong men smoke, some drink coffee, or even liquor, most of them did not have these habits during the years while they wore building their weight, strength and muscle. When they became strong enough such habits were less harmful. You can take your choice, swear off all harmful habits and progress more rapidly, or greatly moderate such habits and retard your progress a great deal less, I am fortunate in the fact that I do not drink anything but water, lemonade or a bit of milk, I never liked coffee, didn't care particularly for tea, never learned to smoke for I was happy enough without it, could not learn to like alcoholic beverages even to the extent of drinking a glass of beer to be polite when invited, have always had good eating habits, and have been rewarded with most unusual health. Not a headache, a sick stomach, or any sort of physical irregularity since I was a child. Have not taken a laxative or needed one since childhood days. This unusual health, exceptional endurance and recuperative powers have given me greater resistance to disease and have made me a leading contender for the title, world's healthiest man. We can't have everything in this world and we obtain most from life by being moderate in all things.

If you really enjoy drinking alcoholic beverages, if you like to smoke, or drink coffee, proper exercise will make it possible for you to live more fully. But if you place your desire to build your body, to acquire more strength, to look better and to feel better, at the head of the list, then you will gain more rapidly and more fully if you eliminate all "leaks," all harmful habits or at least reduce them to the barest minimum.

Back to the important subject of foods. Exercise, in conjunction with right eating, will make important internal changes, improvements in metabolism, digestion, assimilation and elimination. Most important of all, however, is to supply the body with the foods it needs for heat and energy, to rebuild broken down tissue and there must be a surplus with which to build. Some men are naturally blessed with a good digestive and assimilative system, or else habits in earlier life have made it possible for them to build more powerful internal processes. It is easy for such men to make gains. Just supply the body with the food it needs for maintenance and building, just exercise intelligently and intensively, and the gain of the desired poundages is sure to be obtained. But the man who does not have this superior internal strength has a greater task at hand. He must remember that the more laws of health he follows, the fewer omissions and commissions which are a part of his daily life, the more rapid and the better will be his progress.

To make a gain in body weight, first the cells of the body must grow, and they only grow when they are fed the materials they require. Any form of effort-lifting, walking or sex expression, uses up a great deal of the materials the blood has obtained from the food you eat. Therefore it is evident that you can not increase in weight through the increase in size and strength of your muscular fibres unless you not only provide them with sufficient nourishment, vitamins, minerals, chemicals and other elements which supply heat and energy, to supply their general needs but also for an amount to aid in the increase of muscular growth. Making demands upon the muscles, first of all breaking down tissue, supplying the body and the blood with the building materials it requires, is the only means to cause this additional growth and to provide the weight and increases of measurement that are desired.

Exercise such as is offered in this book breaks down tissue, creates demands and progress is made as nature not only meets those demands on the rest days, but produces and stores a bit more as a reserve, to perform even greater tasks when the demand is made. Thus progress is made with progressive training such as is outlined in this course. Make heavier demands upon the body, meet these demands with good food and proper periods of rest, while observing the laws of health, and the physical desires you crave are met.

If you are one who desires to build extra pounds you will need more than fruits and salads, you will need more than fats or starches; you'll need plenty of good solid food, a good share of which will consist of animal protein, milk, eggs, cheese, muscle meat, and some of the glandular meats such as liver, heart, kidneys or pancreas. Particular emphasis should be placed upon the eating of proteins for that is the material of which our bodies are made. We must have protein in ample, properly prepared quantities to build the desired weight and muscle.

BE serious about this planning for a better, more healthful figure. Remember that you have but one body, you'll never get another one. Take care of it, for that body is you, and when some part of it gives out, your life is greatly restricted or ended, depending upon the importance of the worn out part. You must learn how to treat yourself right. Supply your body with the materials it needs: lots of good fresh foods—meals, vegetables, fruit, roast beef, thick steaks, roast lamb, broiled fish and more chicken, oat plenty of roast chicken, boiled chicken, chicken com soup. You'll quickly get stronger, rounder, larger muscles. Eat calves' liver and other forms of liver, chops, fish roe, boiled pork and sauerkraut with mashed potatoes, thick soups with a variety of ingredients, turtle soup without the spices and with plenty of vegetables. Aside from the meat and vegetables with which you are so familiar you will speed your progress by eating some raisins, figs, nuts, dates, cocoanut, eggs, honey, berries, grapes, fruit juices (lemonade sweetened with honey is the most beneficial drink which could be obtained. I have always consumed considerable quantities of lemonade, as much as two quarts a day in my best athletic days. It's good for you, the drinking lemonade habit will be a good one for you); tomato juice, greens and also salads are needed. While many of these will not build weight, particularly the fruits, fruit juices and salads, they are bodily cleansers and they do provide the minerals and vitamins every cell of the body requires.

During the years in which I climbed the ladder to an undisputed position as the "world's leading physical director", I have received many thousands of letters from readers of Strength and Health magazine and from my own pupils, concerning food. Few of them realize that success in body building can not be had without correct eating. Although they complained about their aches, their indigestion, their constipation, they did not know that improper eating was back of most of their difficulty. They took their eating for granted, thought that anything would do just so it was filling, and many of them did not gain as rapidly as they should have. One must remember that the body can not be built any more than a building can be constructed without supplying it with the proper materials. Stone, steel, bricks, mortar, iron and many other materials are needed to build a modern office building. Using poor materials to construct the building means that someday the building will greatly deteriorate, possibly collapse with great loss of life. And if you don't build your own body properly while there is no danger of great loss of life, there is a great danger of the loss of your own life, the life that is most important to you. Make a point to eat proper food and you will be strong, healthy, happy and successful.

Whether you seek to gain weight or lose weight you must supply your body with a great variety of good foods. If underweight, eat more of the foods which build weight, if overweight eat less of the fat forming foods. But in either event supply your body with a variety of foods so that it will have all the ingredients it requires to healthfully maintain it and to build it.

Foods which build weight more rapidly are: nuts of all sorts, bananas with cream and sugar, ice cream, beans, green with butter, limas, cakes, candy, capon, roasted, cream, dates, doughnuts, Russian, French, mayonnaise dressing, duck, particularly stuffed and roasted, eggs, figs, canned salmon, tuna, fish in oils such as sardines, particularly, frankfurters on buttered roll, goose and other fowls, baked egg plant, ham, honey, hot cross bun, jams, jellies, lard, dried lentils, lobster a la Newburg, macaroni with cheese, maple sugar and maple syrup, margarine, marmalade, marshmallow, milk, mincemeat, mutton, olive oil, creamed onions, fried oysters, pancakes with maple syrup, dried pears, dried peas, dried peppers, pineapple with cheese, pears with peanut butter, plum cake, pop corn with butter, all sorts of pork products, potatoes, particularly fried or crisp, preserves, prunes, quince, raisins, most sandwiches, sausage, thick soups, strawberry shortcake, sugar, granulated, highest in caloric content of all, tapioca, tartar sauce, roasted turkey, waffles with syrup, candied yams, zwieback.

Foods which should be included in the reducer's diet in greater quantity, owing to their valuable mineral and vitamin content, of which every person should receive a fair supply, are: apples in most forms, although apple fritters, dumplings and those baked with cream are quite rich, but the apples alone do not build weight, artichokes, asparagus, bananas (contain only 115 calories per portion in spite of the thought most persons have that they are very fat forming), barley soup, canned green beans, raw string beans, only 25 calories, as compared to 425 for navy beans, broccoli, Brussels sprouts, cabbage in any form except with ham or corned beef, cantaloupe, carrots, cauliflower, cranberries, but as sauce contain 225 calories, cucumbers, currants, dandelion, plain eggplant, flounder, bass and cod, contain just

105 calories as compared to 340 for mackerel, fruit salad plain, grapefruit juice, grapes, beet greens, guava, hominy cooked has 80 calories, honeydew melon, huckleberries, ices, kale, kohlrabi only 15 calories, kumquats, leeks, lemons, lettuce, limes, loganberries, mangoes, mushrooms, muskmelon, mussels, noodle soup, 35 calories, okra, onion soup, 50 calories, oranges, raw oysters, papaya, parsley, parsnips, peaches, pears, peas, peppers, pickles, pineapples, plums, potatoes boiled 115, quince, radishes, raspberries, rhubarb, rutabagas, bouillon soup, only 15 calories, spaghetti only 65, spinach, squash, strawberries, Swiss chard, tangerines, tomatoes, turnips, vegetable salad without oil or mayonnaise, watercress, watermelon. The majority of foods in this last group will cause a weight reduction rather than a gain if eaten in quantity, because more calories are required to digest, assimilate and eliminate them than they contain.

HOFFMAN CHART OF WEIGHT AND HEIGHT FOR MEN

Age Groups

Height in feet and inches	20-30			40			50-60		
	H	N	L	H	N	L	H	N	L
5'	120	110	100	125	115	105	121	110	100
5'1"	126	116	105	131	121	110	127	116	105
5'2"	132	122	110	137	127	115	133	122	110
5'3"	140	128	115	145	133	120	141	128	115
5'4"	148	135	121	153	140	126	149	134	120
5'5"	156	141	127	162	147	132	157	140	126
5'6"	165	147	132	171	153	138	165	146	131
5'7"	173	154	138	179	160	144	173	153	137
5'8"	181	160	144	187	166	150	181	159	143
5'9"	189	167	150	195	173	156	189	166	149
5'10"	197	174	156	204	181	162	196	172	155
5'11"	205	181	162	212	188	168	204	179	161
6'	213	188	168	220	195	174	211	185	167
6'1"	221	195	174	228	202	180	219	193	173
6'2"	230	202	180	237	209	186	227	199	179
6'3"	239	208	186	246	215	192	235	204	185

www.ingramcontent.com/pod-product-compliance
Lightning Source LLC
Chambersburg PA
CBHW070215290526
45789CB00002B/994